LOW POTASSIUM DIET COOKBOOK FOR SENIORS

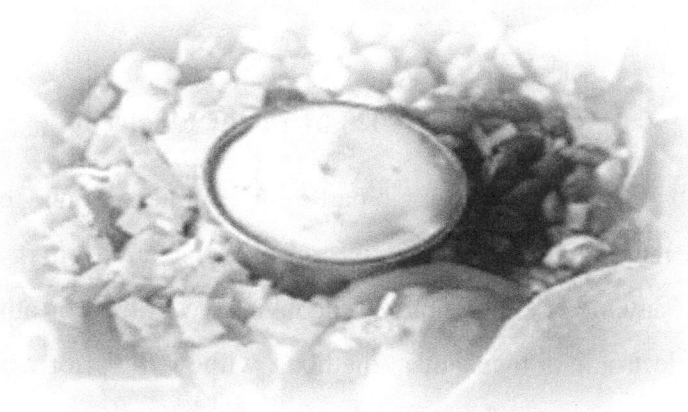

Healthy and Delicious Homemade Recipes to Manage Hyperkalemia and Chronic Kidney Disease

David T. Salcedo

Copyright © 2023 by David T. Salcedo

All rights reserved. No part of this publication may be reproduced, distributed, or transmitted in any form or by any means, including photocopying, recording, or other electronic or mechanical methods, without the prior written permission of the publisher, except in the case of brief quotations embodied in critical reviews and certain other noncommercial uses permitted by copyright law

Table of Contents

INTRODUCTION 5
What is Potassium 8
   Function of Potassium in the Body 8
   Why seniors may need to limit their potassium intake ..11
   Potential health risks of high potassium levels 14
   Common health conditions that require low potassium diets 17
Importance of Low Potassium diet to seniors 21
High Potassium Food to Limit or Avoid 25
CHAPTER 1 28
   Breakfast Recipes 28
CHAPTER 2 38
   Lunch Recipes 38
CHAPTER 3 54
   Dinner Recipes 54
CHAPTER 4 68
   Snacks Recipes 68
CHAPTER 5 77
   Smoothies Recipes 77
CHAPTER 6 87
   7 Days Meal Plan 87
      Day 1 87

Day 2	87
Day 3	87
Day 4	87
Day 5	88
Day 6	88
Day 7	88
CHAPTER 7	89
Conclusion	89

INTRODUCTION

I was confronted with a daunting challenge that would put my resilience and drive to the test. I was diagnosed with chronic kidney disease (CKD), a condition that threatened to derail my previously successful life. I had no idea that this diagnosis would send me on a life-changing path toward better health and a revitalized sense of purpose.

The trip began with a routine examination at my doctor's office, where I learned of my CKD diagnosis. I was overwhelmed with apprehension, worry, and a plethora of questions. My kidneys were no longer functioning properly, according to the doctor, and controlling my potassium levels was critical to delaying the disease's progression.

When I realized this was the case, I knew I needed to make some significant changes in my life. My first step was to adopt a low potassium diet, which looked overwhelming at first. I had to relearn how to purchase, cook, and enjoy food while also monitoring my potassium intake.

Armed with knowledge, I immersed myself in learning about potassium and its effects on my kidneys. I learned how to read food labels, identify high-potassium foods, and look for low-potassium substitutes. This newfound knowledge enabled me to take charge of my health.

The gastronomic adventure that my voyage brought me to was one of the most surprising aspects of my journey. I started experimenting with low potassium meals, learning about new flavors and ingredients along the way. I discovered delight in the kitchen again, making anything from low-potassium smoothies to kidney-friendly casseroles.

Navigating CKD and a low potassium diet can be a lonely process, but I quickly met a community of like-minded people who were also on this trip. Support groups and internet forums gave me vital advice, support, and a feeling of community, which helped me stay motivated.

My health has improved dramatically over the years. My potassium levels stabilized, and the course of my CKD was greatly halted. The trip was not without its difficulties, but with determination and the help of my healthcare team, I overcame adversity.

I discovered a newfound sense of purpose as I restored my health. I became a kidney health advocate, sharing my experience and information with others who were going through similar difficulties. My adventure had not only physically but also emotionally and spiritually transformed me.

Today, I am living proof of the transforming impact of a low potassium diet in the management of chronic renal disease. My path has been one of perseverance, education, and empowerment. It serves as a reminder that, no matter what hurdles we face, we can overcome and thrive with determination and the correct support.

My aim is that my tale may motivate others to pursue improved renal health and a brighter future. Remember, it's never too late to take charge of your health and embark on a new chapter in your life, like I did.

What is Potassium

Potassium (K) is a chemical element with the periodic table symbol "K". It is an essential macromineral, which means that the body needs a lot of it to function effectively. Potassium can be found in a variety of foods, including fruits, vegetables, whole grains, nuts, and seeds. It is also available as a supplement for people who need to enhance their potassium consumption for medical reasons.

Function of Potassium in the Body

Electrolyte Balance: Potassium, along with sodium, calcium, and magnesium, is one of the major electrolytes in the body. These electrolytes aid in the maintenance of cell electrical equilibrium, which is necessary for nerve impulses, muscle contractions, and normal heart rhythm.

Nerve Function: Potassium is necessary for the regular functioning of nerve cells. It aids in the transmission of electrical signals throughout the nervous system, allowing for sensory perception, motor control, and cell communication.

Muscle Function: For healthy contractions, muscle cells, particularly those in the skeletal muscles and the heart (cardiac muscle), need on potassium. A sufficient potassium level is required for muscle strength, coordination, and the prevention of muscle weakness or cramping.

Heart Health: Potassium is essential for controlling the electrical impulses that control the heartbeat. It aids in the maintenance of a stable and regular cardiac rhythm. A lack of potassium (hypokalemia) can cause arrhythmias or irregular heartbeats.

Blood Pressure Regulation: Potassium aids in the regulation of blood pressure by counteracting the effects of sodium. A potassium-rich diet can help reduce blood pressure by relaxing blood vessel walls and decreasing sodium's effect on water retention in the body.

Fluid Balance: Potassium and sodium work together to regulate fluid balance in cells and tissues. It aids in the management of fluid transport into and out of cells, which contributes to general hydration and cellular health.

pH Balance: Potassium ions aid in the maintenance of the body's acid-base balance, which is essential for a variety of metabolic reactions and keeping the pH level within a narrow and healthy range.

Kidney Function: The kidneys are critical in managing potassium levels in the body. They remove extra potassium from the bloodstream and expel it through the urine. Maintaining a healthy potassium balance becomes more difficult in those with renal illness.

Why seniors may need to limit their potassium intake.

Seniors may need to reduce their potassium consumption for a variety of health reasons, particularly if they have specific medical conditions or risk factors. While potassium is vital for numerous body activities, including neuron and muscle function, heart rhythm maintenance, and fluid balance, high potassium levels can be dangerous, especially in older persons. Here are a few reasons why seniors should reduce their potassium intake:

Reduced Kidney Function: Age-related reduction in renal function is one of the most common reasons elders need to limit potassium consumption. The kidneys filter excess potassium from the bloodstream and excrete it in the urine. As people age, their kidney function naturally declines, making it more difficult to maintain healthy potassium levels. This decreased kidney function can result in an increase in potassium levels in the blood, a disease known as hyperkalemia.

Chronic Kidney Disease (CKD): Seniors are more likely to develop chronic kidney disease (CKD), a disorder in which the kidneys gradually lose their ability to filter waste and maintain electrolyte balance. Potassium levels in CKD can become increased, providing a serious health risk. Limiting dietary potassium is an important element of controlling CKD and avoiding problems like irregular heartbeats.

Medication Interactions: Many seniors take medications to treat a variety of health issues. Certain drugs, such as blood pressure medications (e.g., ACE inhibitors and ARBs), can cause a rise in potassium levels in the blood. Seniors using these medications may need to limit their potassium intake to avoid hyperkalemia, which can harm the heart and muscles.

Cardiovascular Health: Seniors are predisposed to cardiovascular problems such as heart disease and hypertension. Elevated potassium levels have the potential to disrupt the electrical signals of the heart, resulting in arrhythmias or irregular heartbeats. Limiting potassium intake in older persons with heart diseases or a history of heart problems can help lower the risk of cardiac consequences.

Reduced Muscle Function: Excess potassium in the blood can impair muscle function, resulting in muscle weakness, cramping, and even paralysis. Seniors who have muscle weakness due to aging or other medical disorders may need to reduce their potassium intake to avoid increasing their symptoms.

Fluid Retention and Edema: Some seniors suffer from fluid retention and edema, which is frequently caused by heart issues or immobility. Foods high in potassium can cause fluid retention by disrupting the sodium-potassium balance in the body. Limiting potassium intake can aid in the management of edema and the maintenance of a healthy fluid balance.

Nutrient Absorption: Due to age-related changes in the digestive tract, seniors may have diminished nutrient absorption. Potassium-rich meals can inhibit the absorption of other vital elements such as calcium and magnesium. Limiting potassium intake can aid in food absorption, which is important for bone health and overall well-being.

Preventing Medication Adjustments: To reduce the need for frequent medication adjustments, especially diuretics and potassium-sparing medications, seniors may be recommended to limit their dietary potassium intake. This helps to keep medications effective while reducing the risk of potassium abnormalities.

Potential health risks of high potassium levels

Hyperkalemia, or high potassium levels in the blood, can be dangerous to one's health. Potassium is an essential element that plays an important part in many biological functions, but when its levels grow extremely high, it can cause a variety of negative health effects. Here are some of the health dangers associated with high potassium levels, along with explanations for each:

Cardiac Arrhythmias: Elevated potassium levels can alter heart electrical signals, resulting in irregular heart beats or arrhythmias. These irregular heartbeats can be fatal, causing palpitations, dizziness, fainting, and, in severe cases, cardiac arrest.

Muscle Weakness: High potassium levels can impair muscular function. It can cause muscle weakness, tiredness, and, in extreme circumstances, paralysis. This can impair a person's ability to carry out everyday tasks and increase the likelihood of falls and injury.

Nausea and Vomiting: Hyperkalemia can cause gastrointestinal symptoms such as nausea, vomiting, and abdominal discomfort. These symptoms can lead to malnutrition and dehydration, especially if they cause a decrease in food and fluid intake.

Breathing Difficulties: In extreme cases of hyperkalemia, respiratory muscles may be damaged, resulting in trouble breathing. This can be quite harmful and necessitates emergency medical intervention.

Heart Palpitations: Hyperkalemia can cause uncomfortable heart palpitations. These irregular heartbeats, which can feel like fluttering or a rapid heartbeat, are frequently accompanied by worry.

Kidney Function Impairment: Over time, chronic hyperkalemia might cause kidney damage. The kidneys are in charge of managing potassium levels in the body, and high potassium levels can strain the kidneys and decrease their capacity to operate effectively.

Increased Risk of Stroke: Some studies suggest a possible link between high potassium levels and an increased risk of stroke, especially in people with specific underlying health conditions. More study, however, is required to definitively confirm this association.

Hypotension (Low Blood Pressure): Hyperkalemia can cause low blood pressure (hypotension) in some people. This can cause dizziness and lightheadedness, as well as an increased risk of falling and fainting.

Metabolic Acidosis: High potassium levels can contribute to metabolic acidosis, which is an imbalance in the body's acid-base equilibrium. This can result in a variety of symptoms such as disorientation, weakness, and changes in breathing patterns.

Complications for Individuals with Kidney Disease: High potassium levels are a significant source of concern for people with chronic kidney disease (CKD). Hyperkalemia can worsen kidney impairment and raise the risk of cardiovascular problems.

Common health conditions that require low potassium diets

A low potassium diet may be required to treat and prevent consequences associated with excessive potassium levels (hyperkalemia) in a variety of health diseases and medical circumstances. It's important to note that potassium limitations can vary depending on the severity of the ailment and individual circumstances. The following are some common health issues that may necessitate a low potassium diet:

Chronic Kidney Disease (CKD)

One of the most common reasons for a low potassium diet is CKD. The kidneys are crucial in controlling potassium levels in the body. As CKD progresses, the kidneys may struggle to eliminate extra potassium, resulting in hyperkalemia. A low potassium diet is critical for potassium management and lowering the risk of heart and muscle problems.

End-Stage Renal Disease (ESRD)

Individuals with end-stage renal disease (ESRD), the most advanced stage of kidney failure, may require dialysis to remove trash and excess potassium from their blood. Potassium levels can fluctuate even with dialysis, and a low potassium diet is usually recommended to reduce the risk of hyperkalemia.

Hypertension (High Blood Pressure)

A low-sodium diet can occasionally be used to manage high blood pressure, which may indirectly lower potassium intake because many high-potassium foods are also high in salt. Controlling potassium intake can assist in maintaining healthy blood pressure levels.

Certain Medications

Some drugs might cause a rise in blood potassium levels. Certain diuretics (potassium-sparing diuretics), ACE inhibitors, angiotensin II receptor blockers (ARBs), and nonsteroidal anti-inflammatory medications (NSAIDs) may be among them. Individuals taking these drugs may need to reduce their dietary potassium intake in order to avoid hyperkalemia.

Addison's Disease

Addison's disease is an uncommon disorder characterized by insufficient adrenal hormone production. It can lead to electrolyte abnormalities, especially potassium. Dietary potassium management may be required as part of the therapy regimen.

Acute Kidney Injury (AKI)

Temporary kidney malfunction in cases of acute kidney injury can result in electrolyte abnormalities, particularly potassium. To avoid difficulties during the recovery period, a low potassium diet may be advised.

Gastrointestinal Disorders

Excess potassium loss can be caused by gastrointestinal diseases such as prolonged diarrhea or malabsorption problems. In such circumstances, a low potassium diet may be advised to avoid potassium deficiency.

Heart Conditions

To lower the risk of arrhythmias and other cardiac problems, some heart disorders, particularly those affecting the electrical activity of the heart, may necessitate potassium limits.

Post-Kidney Transplant

Individuals who have had a kidney transplant may need to follow a low potassium diet for a while as the donated kidney adjusts to its new function. Dietary restrictions may be relaxed with time, but potassium intake must still be monitored.

Importance of Low Potassium diet to seniors

A low potassium diet is critical for seniors, especially those with chronic kidney disease (CKD) or other underlying health disorders that influence renal function. Potassium is a mineral that is required for many body activities, including neuron and muscle function, appropriate heart rhythm, and fluid balance. However, for seniors, striking the appropriate potassium balance becomes critical for various reasons:

Kidney Function Declines with Age

Kidney function naturally declines as people age. The kidneys are in charge of filtering excess potassium from the bloodstream. When kidney function declines, the body may struggle to adequately manage potassium levels, potentially leading to a buildup of potassium in the blood (hyperkalemia).

A low potassium diet eases the stress on aging kidneys, making potassium levels easier to maintain.

Managing Chronic Kidney Disease (CKD)

Chronic kidney disease, which can grow gradually for years before symptoms arise, is more common in seniors. The kidneys' ability to filter waste and maintain potassium.

To prevent hyperkalemia, which can lead to deadly cardiac arrhythmias, a low potassium diet is frequently advised as part of the treatment strategy for CKD homeostasis is impaired in CKD.

Reducing the Risk of Cardiovascular Complications

High potassium levels in the blood can harm the cardiovascular system, increasing the risk of heart palpitations, abnormal heart rhythms, and even sudden cardiac arrest.

Seniors, who are already at a higher risk of heart disease, benefit from a low potassium diet to help them avoid these difficulties.

Medication Interactions

Seniors may be on a variety of drugs to treat chronic health concerns. Certain drugs, such as blood pressure medications (ACE inhibitors and ARBs), can cause an increase in potassium levels in the blood.

A low potassium diet helps to offset these drugs' potassium-raising effects, lowering the risk of hyperkalemia.

Management of Fluid Balance

Fluid retention is also a problem for seniors due to a variety of reasons such as restricted mobility, certain medications, and heart-related diseases. A low potassium diet can aid in fluid balance management by restricting the consumption of foods high in both potassium and sodium, both of which contribute to fluid retention.

Promoting Bone Health

Seniors are more prone to osteoporosis and weak bones. A low potassium diet frequently includes low phosphorus meals, which can assist preserve bone health because high phosphorus levels can leach calcium from bones.

Preventing Muscle Weakness and Fatigue

Excess potassium can cause muscle weakness and weariness. Maintaining muscle strength and function is critical for seniors' everyday activities and overall quality of life.

Improving Overall Nutrition

A low potassium diet supports a well-balanced diet that contains other vital nutrients such as vitamins, minerals, fiber, and protein in addition to limiting potassium intake.

This comprehensive approach to diet can assist seniors by promoting overall health and well-being.

High Potassium Food to Limit or Avoid

Individuals who need to monitor their potassium intake owing to health issues such as chronic kidney disease (CKD), kidney-related diseases, or drugs that might spike potassium levels should avoid high potassium foods. The following foods are high in potassium and should be limited or avoided:

1. *Bananas* are well-known for their high potassium content. A medium-sized banana has 400-450 mg of potassium.

2. *Oranges and Orange Juice*: Oranges and orange juice contain a lot of potassium. A medium-sized orange has about 237 milligrams of potassium.

3. *Potatoes* are abundant in potassium and come in both white and sweet variants. Over 900 mg of potassium can be found in a medium-sized roasted potato with skin.

4. *Tomatoes and tomato-based products* such as tomato sauce, tomato paste, and ketchup are high in potassium. One cup of tomato sauce contains around 900 milligrams of potassium.

5. ***Dried Fruits***: Dried fruits with high potassium levels include raisins, apricots, and prunes. A quarter-cup of raisins has around 270 milligrams of potassium.

6. ***Avocado*** is a nutritious fruit that is also high in potassium. One medium avocado has about 975 milligrams of potassium.

7. ***Spinach*** is high in potassium, as are other leafy greens. One cup of cooked spinach has almost 800 milligrams of potassium.

8. ***Beans and lentils***: Beans (such as kidney beans and black beans) and lentils are high in potassium. A half-cup of cooked kidney beans has around 360 milligrams of potassium.

9. ***Dairy items***: Dairy items such as milk, yogurt, and cheese can help you get enough potassium. Low-fat and nonfat dairy products may be preferable for persons on a low-potassium diet.

10. ***Nuts and Seeds***: Potassium-rich nuts and seeds include almonds, peanuts, and sunflower seeds. A quarter-cup of almonds has about 210 milligrams of potassium.

11. *Fish:* Certain forms of fish, such as salmon and tuna, contain a moderate amount of potassium. While they include vital nutrients, portion control may be required.

12. ***Processed foods***, such as canned soups, processed meats, and convenience foods, may have additional potassium as a preservative or flavor enhancer. Check the potassium content of foods on the label.

13. ***Potassium-Fortified Foods and Drinks***: Be wary of potassium-fortified foods and beverages, as they can considerably contribute to daily intake.

14. ***Potassium chloride*** is used as a sodium replacement in several salt substitutes. Individuals on a low potassium diet should avoid or use them cautiously.

CHAPTER 1

Breakfast Recipes

1. Spinach and Tomato with Scrambled Egg Whites

Ingredients

- 2 egg whites
- 1/2 cup fresh spinach (cooked and drained)
- 1/4 cup diced tomatoes (canned with low potassium content)
- Salt and pepper to taste

Preparation

- The egg should be Whisked in a bowl.
- Add the cooked spinach and diced tomatoes.
- Season with salt and pepper.
- Cook in a non-stick skillet over low heat until the eggs are set.

Nutritional Information

Calories: 70

Protein: 14g

Potassium: 220mg

Preparation Time: 15 minutes

Serving Size: 1

2. Oatmeal with Cinnamon and Apple

Ingredients

- Rolled oats (cooked with water) of ½ Cup
- 1/2 teaspoon cinnamon
- 1/2 small apple, diced (peeled)

Preparation

- Oats should be cooked with water according to package instructions.
- Stir in cinnamon and top with diced apple.

Nutritional Information

- Calories: 150
- Protein: 4g
- Potassium: 110mg

Preparation Time: 10 minutes

Serving Size: 1

3. Greek Yogurt Parfait

Ingredients

- 1/2 cup plain Greek yogurt (low potassium)
- 1/4 cup sliced strawberries
- 1 tablespoon honey (optional)
- 1 tablespoon chopped almonds (in limited quantity)

Preparation

- Layer Greek yogurt, sliced strawberries, honey (if desired), and chopped almonds in a glass or bowl.

Nutritional Information

- Calories: 180
- Protein: 12g
- Potassium: 150mg

Preparation Time: 5 minutes

Serving Size: 1

4. Cottage Cheese and Pineapple Bowl

Ingredients

- 1/2 cup low-fat cottage cheese
- 1/2 cup diced pineapple (canned with low potassium content)
- 1 tablespoon shredded coconut (in limited quantity)

Preparation

- Combine cottage cheese and diced pineapple in a bowl.
- Sprinkle with shredded coconut.

Nutritional Information

- Calories: 150
- Protein: 12g
- Potassium: 180mg

Preparation Time: 5 minutes

Serving Size: 1

5. Rice Cake with Almond Butter and Banana

Ingredients

- 1 rice cake (choose a low potassium brand)
- 1 tablespoon almond butter (in limited quantity)
- 1/2 small banana, sliced

Preparation

- Almond butter should be spread on the rice cake.
- Top with sliced banana.

Nutritional Information

Calories: 150

Protein: 2g

Potassium: 110mg

Preparation Time: 5 minutes

Serving Size: 1

6. Egg and Spinach Breakfast Wrap

Ingredients

- 1 whole wheat tortilla (low potassium)
- 1 boiled egg, sliced
- 1/2 cup fresh spinach (cooked and drained)

Preparation

- Lay the sliced boiled egg and cooked spinach on the tortilla.
- Roll up to make a breakfast wrap.

Nutritional Information

- Calories: 180
- Protein: 12g
- Potassium: 160mg

Preparation Time: 10 minutes

Serving Size: 1

7. Quinoa Breakfast Bowl

Ingredients

- 1/2 cup cooked quinoa
- 1/4 cup sliced strawberries
- 1 tablespoon chopped pecans (in limited quantity)
- 1 teaspoon honey (optional)

Preparation

- Combine cooked quinoa, sliced strawberries, and chopped pecans in a bowl.
- Drizzle with honey if desired.

Nutritional Information

- Calories: 200
- Protein: 4g
- Potassium: 120mg

Preparation Time: 15 minutes

Serving Size: 1

8. Cottage Cheese Pancakes

Ingredients

- 1/2 cup low-fat cottage cheese
- 2 eggs
- 2 tablespoons oat flour (made from low potassium oats)
- 1/2 teaspoon vanilla extract

Preparation

- Blend cottage cheese, eggs, oat flour, and vanilla extract until smooth.
- Cook small pancakes on a non-stick skillet.

Nutritional Information

- Calories: 250
- Protein: 25g
- Potassium: 170mg

Preparation Time: 15 minutes

Serving Size: 1

9. Low Potassium Smoothie

Ingredients

- 1/2 cup unsweetened almond milk (low potassium)
- 1/2 cup frozen berries (e.g., blueberries, raspberries)
- 1/4 cup spinach
- 1 tablespoon chia seeds (in limited quantity)
- 1/2 banana (choose a low potassium brand)

Preparation

- Blend all the ingredients until smooth.

Nutritional Information

Calories: 120

Protein: 3g

Potassium: 150mg

Preparation Time: 5 minutes

Serving Size: 1

10. Cream of Wheat Cereal

Ingredients

- 1/2 cup Cream of Wheat cereal (prepare with water)
- 1/4 cup sliced peaches (canned with low potassium content)
- 1 tablespoon chopped walnuts (in limited quantity)

Preparation

- Cook the Cream of Wheat cereal with water according to package instructions.
- Top with sliced peaches and chopped walnuts.

Nutritional Information

Calories: 180

Protein: 5g

Potassium: 140mg

Preparation Time: 10 minutes

Serving Size: 1

CHAPTER 2

Lunch Recipes

1. Chicken and Vegetable Stir-Fry

Ingredients

- 4 oz (113g) boneless, skinless chicken breast, sliced
- 1 cup broccoli florets
- 1/2 cup red bell pepper, sliced
- 1/2 cup snow peas
- 1 tablespoon low-sodium soy sauce
- 1 teaspoon minced garlic
- 1 teaspoon sesame oil
- 1 tablespoon canola oil
- Cooked white rice (optional)

Preparation

- The canola oil should be heated in a pan over medium-high heat.
- Chicken should be added and cooked until no longer pink.
- Add vegetables, garlic, and soy sauce. Stir-fry until vegetables are tender.

- Drizzle with sesame oil.
- Serve over cooked white rice if desired.

Nutritional Information

- Calories: 300
- Protein: 25g
- Carbohydrates: 16g
- Fiber: 3g
- Potassium: 300mg

Preparation Time: 20 minutes

Serving Size: 1

2. Quinoa and Black Bean Salad

Ingredients

- 1 cup cooked quinoa
- 1/2 cup canned black beans (rinsed and drained)
- 1/4 cup diced red onion
- 1/4 cup diced cucumber
- 1/4 cup diced red bell pepper
- 2 tablespoons chopped fresh cilantro
- 1 tablespoon olive oil
- 1 tablespoon fresh lime juice
- Salt and pepper to taste

Preparation

- In a bowl, combine quinoa, black beans, red onion, cucumber, red bell pepper, and cilantro.
- In a separate bowl, whisk together olive oil and lime juice. Season with salt and pepper.
- The dressing should be drizzled over the salad and toss to combine.

Nutritional Information

Calories: 230

Protein: 7g

Carbohydrates: 34g

Fiber: 7g

Potassium: 210mg

Preparation Time: 15 minutes

Serving Size: 1

3. Turkey and Vegetable Wrap

Ingredients

- 2 oz (56g) low-sodium turkey breast slices
- 1 whole wheat tortilla
- 1/4 cup lettuce leaves
- 1/4 cup sliced cucumber
- 1/4 cup sliced red bell pepper
- 1 tablespoon low-sodium hummus

Preparation

- The tortilla should be laid flat and spread hummus evenly.
- Place turkey slices, lettuce, cucumber, and red bell pepper on the tortilla.
- Roll up the tortilla tightly.

Nutritional Information

- Calories: 250
- Protein: 16g
- Carbohydrates: 30g
- Fiber: 6g
- Potassium: 200mg

Preparation Time: 10 minutes

Serving Size: 1

4. Spinach and Mushroom Omelette

Ingredients

- 2 large eggs
- 1/4 cup chopped spinach
- 1/4 cup sliced mushrooms
- 2 tablespoons diced onion
- 1/2 tablespoon canola oil
- Salt and pepper to taste

Preparation

- The eggs should be beaten in a bowl and seasoned with salt and pepper.
- Canola oil should be heated in a non-stick skillet over medium heat.
- Onions and mushrooms should be added, sauté until tender.
- The beaten eggs should be poured over the vegetables and cook until set.
- Omelette should be folded in half and serve.

Nutritional Information

- Calories: 180
- Protein: 12g
- Carbohydrates: 4g
- Fiber: 1g
- Potassium: 150mg

Preparation Time: 15 minutes

Serving Size: 1

5. Tuna and White Bean Salad

Ingredients

- Canned white beans (rinsed and drained) of 1/2 cup
- 3 oz (85g) canned tuna (packed in water, drained)
- 1/4 cup diced celery
- 1/4 cup diced red onion
- 1 tablespoon lemon juice
- 1 tablespoon olive oil
- Salt and pepper to taste

Preparation

- In a bowl, combine white beans, tuna, celery, and red onion.
- In a separate bowl, whisk together lemon juice and olive oil. Season with salt and pepper.
- The dressing should be drizzled over the salad and toss to combine.

Nutritional Information

- Calories: 280
- Protein: 22g
- Carbohydrates: 19g
- Fiber: 5g
- Potassium: 320mg

Preparation Time: 10 minutes

Serving Size: 1

6. Broccoli and Rice Casserole

Ingredients

- 1 cup cooked white rice
- 1 cup chopped broccoli (cooked)
- 1/4 cup grated low-sodium cheddar cheese
- 2 tablespoons plain Greek yogurt
- 1/2 teaspoon garlic powder
- Salt and pepper to taste

Preparation

- Preheat the oven to 350°F (175°C).
- In a mixing bowl, combine cooked rice, chopped broccoli, grated cheddar cheese, Greek yogurt, garlic powder, salt, and pepper.
- The mixture should be transferred to a baking dish.
- It should be baked for 15-20 minutes or until the cheese is melted and bubbly.

Nutritional Information

- Calories: 270
- Protein: 10g
- Carbohydrates: 45g
- Fiber: 3g
- Potassium: 280mg

Preparation Time: 30 minutes

Serving Size: 1

7. Grilled Chicken Salad with Lemon Dressing

Ingredients

- 4 oz (113g) grilled chicken breast, sliced
- 2 cups mixed greens (e.g., lettuce, arugula, spinach)
- 1/4 cup cherry tomatoes, halved
- 1/4 cup sliced cucumber
- 1/4 cup sliced red onion
- 1 tablespoon olive oil
- 1 tablespoon fresh lemon juice
- Salt and pepper to taste

Preparation

- Combine the following in a large bowl Cherry tomatoes, cucumber, mixed greens and red onion.
- Top with grilled chicken slices.
- Olive oil, lemon juice, salt, and pepper should be whisked in a small bowl.
- Drizzle over the salad.

Nutritional Information

- Calories: 290
- Protein: 27g
- Carbohydrates: 9g
- Fiber: 3g
- Potassium: 250mg

Preparation Time: 20 minutes

Serving Size: 1

8. Eggplant and Tomato Bake

Ingredients

- 1 small eggplant, sliced
- 1 cup sliced tomatoes
- 2 tablespoons olive oil
- 1/2 teaspoon dried basil
- 1/2 teaspoon dried oregano
- 1/4 cup grated low-sodium mozzarella cheese

Preparation

- Preheat the oven to 375°F (190°C).
- In a baking dish, arrange slices of eggplant and tomatoes in alternating layers.
- Drizzle with olive oil and sprinkle with dried basil and oregano.
- Top with grated mozzarella cheese.
- The vegetables should be baked for 25-30 minutes until its tender and the cheese is golden brown.

Nutritional Information

- Calories: 220
- Protein: 6g
- Carbohydrates: 15g
- Fiber: 6g
- Potassium: 230mg

Preparation Time: 35 minutes

Serving Size: 1

9. Turkey and Vegetable Soup

Ingredients

- 2 cups low-sodium chicken broth
- 2 oz (56g) cooked turkey breast, diced
- 1/2 cup diced carrots
- 1/2 cup diced celery
- 1/2 cup diced zucchini
- 1/4 cup diced onion
- 1/2 teaspoon dried thyme
- Salt and pepper to taste

Preparation

- In a pot, combine chicken broth, diced turkey, carrots, celery, zucchini, onion, dried thyme, salt, and pepper.
- Vegetables should be brought to a boil, reduce heat and simmer for 15-20 minutes or until its tender.

Nutritional Information

- Calories: 160
- Protein: 16g
- Carbohydrates: 12g
- Fiber: 2g
- Potassium: 270mg

Preparation Time: 30 minutes

Serving Size: 1

10. Baked Salmon with Lemon and Herbs

Ingredients

- 4 oz (113g) salmon fillet
- 1 tablespoon fresh lemon juice
- 1/2 teaspoon dried dill
- 1/2 teaspoon dried parsley
- Salt and pepper to taste

Preparation

- Preheat the oven to 375°F (190°C).
- The salmon fillet should be placed on a baking sheet.
- Drizzle with fresh lemon juice and sprinkle with dried dill, dried parsley, salt, and pepper.
- It should be baked for 15-20 minutes or until the salmon flakes easily with a fork.

Nutritional Information

- Calories: 220
- Protein: 23g
- Carbohydrates: 1g
- Fiber: 0g
- Potassium: 300mg

Preparation Time: 20 minutes

Serving Size: 1

CHAPTER 3

Dinner Recipes

1. Lemon Herb Baked Chicken

Ingredients

- 4 boneless, skinless chicken breasts
- 2 lemons, sliced
- 2 tsp olive oil
- 1 tsp dried rosemary
- 1 tsp dried thyme
- Salt and pepper to taste

Preparation

- Preheat the oven to 375°F (190°C).
- Season chicken breasts with salt, pepper, rosemary, and thyme.
- Lemon slices should be placed on top of each chicken breast.
- Drizzle with olive oil.
- Bake for 25-30 minutes until the chicken is cooked through.

Nutritional Information

- Potassium: Approximately 150mg
- Protein: 30g

Prep Time: 10 minutes

Serving Size: 1 chicken breast

2. Quinoa and Vegetable Stir-Fry

Ingredients

- 1 cup quinoa, uncooked
- 2 cups low-sodium vegetable broth
- Mixed vegetables (e.g., bell peppers, broccoli, carrots) of 2 Cups.
- 2 tbsp low-sodium soy sauce
- 1 tbsp olive oil
- 1 clove garlic, minced

Preparation

- Rinse quinoa under cold water.
- Quinoa and vegetable broth should be combined in a saucepan.
- It should be brought to a boil, then reduce heat and simmer for 15-20 minutes.
- In a separate pan, sauté mixed vegetables in olive oil and garlic.
- Mix cooked quinoa with sautéed vegetables and soy sauce.

Nutritional Information

- Potassium: Approximately 200mg
- Protein: 8g

Prep Time: 10 minutes

Serving Size: 1 cup

3. Baked Cod with Herbed Cauliflower Rice

Ingredients

- 4 cod fillets
- 1 head cauliflower, grated
- 2 tbsp fresh parsley, chopped
- 2 tbsp fresh dill, chopped
- 2 tbsp lemon juice
- 1 tbsp olive oil
- Salt and pepper to taste

Preparation

- Preheat the oven to 375°F (190°C).
- Cod fillets should be seasoned with salt, pepper, and lemon juice. Place them in a baking dish.
- In a separate bowl, mix grated cauliflower, parsley, dill, and olive oil.
- Spread the cauliflower mixture over the cod.
- It should be baked for 20-25 minutes until the fish flakes easily.

Nutritional Information

- Potassium: Approximately 250mg
- Protein: 30g

Cooking Time: 25 minutes

Serving Size: 1 cod fillet with cauliflower rice

4. Spinach and Mushroom Stuffed Chicken Breast

Ingredients

- 4 boneless, skinless chicken breasts
- 2 cups spinach, chopped
- 1 cup mushrooms, sliced
- 2 cloves garlic, minced
- 1/4 cup low-sodium chicken broth
- 1/4 cup low-fat mozzarella cheese
- Salt and pepper to taste

Preparation

- Preheat the oven to 375°F (190°C).
- In a skillet, sauté mushrooms and garlic in chicken broth until tender.
- Chopped spinach should be stirred and cook until wilted.
- Make a pocket in each chicken breast and stuff with the spinach-mushroom mixture.
- Season chicken with salt and pepper, then sprinkle with mozzarella cheese.
- It should be baked for 25-30 minutes until chicken is cooked through and cheese is melted.

Nutritional Information

- Potassium: Approximately 200mg
- Protein: 30g

Prep Time: 15 minutes

Serving Size: 1 stuffed chicken breast

5. Turkey and Vegetable Stir-Fry

Ingredients

- 1 lb lean ground turkey
- 2 cups mixed vegetables (e.g., bell peppers, snow peas, carrots)
- 2 tbsp low-sodium soy sauce
- 1 tbsp olive oil
- 1 tsp ginger, minced
- 1 tsp garlic, minced

Preparation

- In a skillet, heat olive oil and sauté ginger and garlic until fragrant.
- Ground turkey should be added and cook until browned.
- Stir in mixed vegetables and soy sauce. Cook until vegetables are tender.

Nutritional Information

- Potassium: Approximately 250mg
- Protein: 25g

Prep Time: 10 minutes

Serving Size: Approximately 1 cup

6. Lentil and Vegetable Soup

Ingredients

- 1 cup green lentils, rinsed
- 4 cups low-sodium vegetable broth
- 2 cups mixed vegetables (e.g., carrots, celery, zucchini)
- 1 tsp olive oil
- 1 tsp cumin
- Salt and pepper to taste

Preparation

- Heat olive oil in a large pot and sauté mixed vegetables until softened.
- Add lentils, vegetable broth, cumin, salt, and pepper.
- Simmer for 25-30 minutes until lentils are tender.

Nutritional Information

- Potassium: Approximately 300mg
- Protein: 10g

Prep Time: 10 minutes

Serving Size: Approximately 1 cup

7. Salmon and Asparagus Foil Packets

Ingredients

- 4 salmon fillets
- 2 bunches asparagus, trimmed
- 2 tbsp lemon juice
- 2 tsp olive oil
- Fresh dill for garnish
- Salt and pepper to taste

Preparation

- Preheat the oven to 375°F (190°C).
- The salmon fillet should be placed on a piece of aluminum foil.
- Arrange asparagus around the salmon.
- Drizzle lemon juice and olive oil over the salmon and asparagus.
- It should be seasoned with salt, pepper, and fresh dill.
- Seal the foil packets and bake for 20-25 minutes until salmon is cooked.

Nutritional Information

- Potassium: Approximately 250mg
- Protein: 30g

Prep Time: 10 minutes

Serving Size: 1 salmon fillet with asparagus

8. Eggplant Parmesan

Ingredients

- 2 medium eggplants, sliced into rounds
- 1 cup low-sodium tomato sauce
- 1/2 cup part-skim mozzarella cheese
- 1/4 cup grated Parmesan cheese
- 1/4 cup fresh basil, chopped
- 1 tsp olive oil
- Salt and pepper to taste

Preparation

- Preheat the oven to 375°F (190°C).
- The eggplant slices should be brushed with olive oil and season with salt and pepper.
- Bake eggplant slices for 20-25 minutes until tender.
- In a baking dish, layer eggplant slices with tomato sauce, mozzarella cheese, and Parmesan cheese.
- Repeat layers and bake for an additional 20-25 minutes until cheese is bubbly.
- Garnish with fresh basil.

Nutritional Information

- Potassium: Approximately 300mg
- Protein: 10g

Prep Time: 20 minutes

Serving Size: 2 eggplant slices

9. Turkey and Vegetable Skewers

Ingredients

- 1 lb lean ground turkey
- Mixed vegetables (e.g., bell peppers, zucchini, cherry tomatoes) of 2 cups.
- 2 tbsp low-sodium soy sauce
- 1 tsp olive oil
- 1 tsp dried oregano
- Salt and pepper to taste

Preparation

- Preheat the grill or grill pan.
- In a bowl, mix ground turkey with soy sauce, olive oil, oregano, salt, and pepper.
- Form turkey mixture into small meatballs.

- Meatballs and mixed vegetables should be threaded onto skewers.
- Grill skewers for 10-12 minutes, turning occasionally, until turkey is cooked and vegetables are tender.

Nutritional Information

- Potassium: Approximately 250mg
- Protein: 20g

Prep Time: 15 minutes

Serving Size: 2 skewers

10. Tofu and Broccoli Stir-Fry

Ingredients

- 1 block extra-firm tofu, cubed
- 2 cups broccoli florets
- 2 tbsp low-sodium soy sauce
- 1 tbsp sesame oil
- 1 tsp ginger, minced
- 1 tsp garlic, minced
- Salt and pepper to taste

Preparation

- In a wok or large skillet, heat sesame oil and sauté ginger and garlic until fragrant.
- Cubed tofu should be added and cook until lightly browned.
- Stir in broccoli florets and soy sauce. Cook until broccoli is tender.
- Season with salt and pepper.

Nutritional Information

- Potassium: Approximately 200mg
- Protein: 15g

Prep Time: 15 minutes

Serving Size: Approximately 1 cup

CHAPTER 4

Snacks Recipes

1. Cucumber and Cottage Cheese Bites

Ingredients

- 1 medium cucumber, sliced into rounds
- 1/2 cup low-fat cottage cheese
- Fresh dill (optional, for garnish)

Preparation

- Spread a small amount of cottage cheese on each cucumber round.
- Garnish with fresh dill if desired.
- Serve chilled.

Nutritional Information

- Calories: 50
- Protein: 6g
- Carbohydrates: 4g
- Fat: 1g
- Potassium: 60mg

Preparation Time: 10 minutes

2. Rice Cake with Peanut Butter

Ingredients

- 1 rice cake (low sodium)
- 1 tablespoon unsalted peanut butter

Preparation

- Spread peanut butter over the rice cake.
- It should be served as a crunchy and satisfying snack.

Nutritional Information

- Calories: 80
- Protein: 2g
- Carbohydrates: 7g
- Fat: 5g
- Potassium: 50mg

Preparation Time: 2 minutes

3. Baked Sweet Potato Fries

Ingredients

- 1 small sweet potato, cut into fries
- 1 teaspoon olive oil
- Seasonings (e.g., paprika, garlic powder, rosemary, optional)

Preparation

- Sweet potato fries should be tossed with olive oil and seasonings.
- Spread on a baking sheet and bake at 400°F (200°C) for 20-25 minutes until crispy.
- Let cool slightly before serving.

Nutritional Information

- Calories: 70
- Protein: 1g
- Carbohydrates: 16g
- Fat: 1g
- Potassium: 100mg

Preparation Time: 35 minutes

4. Celery Sticks with Hummus

Ingredients

- 2 celery sticks, cut into snack-sized pieces
- 2 tablespoons low-potassium hummus

Preparation

- Spread hummus on celery sticks.
- Enjoy this crunchy and protein-rich snack.

Nutritional Information

- Calories: 50
- Protein: 2g
- Carbohydrates: 4g
- Fat: 3g
- Potassium: 140mg

Preparation Time: 5 minutes

5. Cottage Cheese with Pineapple

Ingredients

- 1/2 cup low-fat cottage cheese
- Canned pineapple tidbits (in juice, drained) of 1/4 cup
- A sprinkle of cinnamon (optional)

Preparation

- Mix cottage cheese and pineapple together.
- Cinnamon dash should be added for extra flavor, if desired.
- Serve chilled.

Nutritional Information

- Calories: 130
- Protein: 14g
- Carbohydrates: 16g
- Fat: 2g
- Potassium: 190mg

Preparation Time: 5 minutes

6. Apple Slices with Almond Butter

Ingredients

- 1 small apple, sliced
- 1 tablespoon unsalted almond butter

Preparation

- Spread almond butter on apple slices.
- Enjoy the combination of crisp apples and creamy almond butter.

Nutritional Information

- Calories: 150
- Protein: 2g
- Carbohydrates: 23g
- Fat: 7g
- Potassium: 175mg

Preparation Time: 3 minutes

7. Tuna Salad Lettuce Wraps

Ingredients

- 1/2 cup canned tuna (packed in water, drained)
- 1 tablespoon low-potassium mayonnaise
- 1 teaspoon mustard
- Lettuce leaves (e.g., iceberg, Romaine)

Preparation

- In a bowl, mix tuna, mayonnaise, and mustard until well combined.
- The tuna salad should be spooned onto lettuce leaves and wrap them up.
- Enjoy as a protein-packed snack.

Nutritional Information

- Calories: 160
- Protein: 17g
- Carbohydrates: 2g
- Fat: 10g
- Potassium: 160mg

Preparation Time: 5 minutes

8. Low-Potassium Vegetable Crudité

Ingredients

- Assorted low-potassium vegetables (e.g., carrots, cucumber, bell peppers)
- Low-potassium ranch or yogurt-based dip

Preparation

- Wash, peel, and cut the vegetables into bite-sized sticks or pieces.
- Serve with a side of low-potassium dip for added flavor.

Nutritional Information

- Calories: Varies based on vegetables and dip
- Protein: Varies
- Carbohydrates: Varies
- Fat: Varies
- Potassium: Varies

Preparation Time: 10 minutes

9. Rice Cake with Sliced Strawberries

Ingredients

- 1 rice cake (low sodium)
- 1/4 cup sliced strawberries
- 1 tablespoon low-potassium whipped topping (optional)

Preparation

- Top the rice cake with sliced strawberries.
- For added indulgence, add a dollop of low-potassium whipped topping.
- Enjoy this sweet and satisfying snack.

Nutritional Information

- Calories: 40
- Protein: 0.5g
- Carbohydrates: 9g
- Fat: 0g
- Potassium: 35mg

Preparation Time: 2 minutes

CHAPTER 5

Smoothies Recipes

1. Berry Blast Smoothie

Ingredients

- 1/2 cup blueberries (low in potassium)
- 1/2 cup strawberries (low in potassium)
- 1/2 banana (sliced, remove potassium by soaking in water)
- 1/2 cup low-potassium yogurt
- 1/2 cup unsweetened almond milk (or low-potassium milk substitute)
- 1 tbsp honey (optional)

Preparation

- Combine all ingredients in a blender.
- Blend until smooth.

Nutritional Information

- Calories: 180
- Protein: 6g
- Potassium: Approximately 130mg

Serving Size: 1 smoothie

Preparation Time: 5 minutes

2. Creamy Green Avocado Smoothie

Ingredients

- 1/4 ripe avocado (peeled and pitted)
- 1/2 cup baby spinach
- 1/2 cup cucumber (peeled and chopped)
- 1/2 cup low-potassium yogurt
- 1/2 cup water
- 1 tsp lemon juice
- Ice cubes (optional)

Preparation

- Place all ingredients in a blender.
- Blend until creamy and smooth.

Nutritional Information

- Calories: 110
- Protein: 3g
- Potassium: Approximately 120mg

Serving Size: 1 smoothie

Preparation Time: 5 minutes

3. Apple Pie Smoothie

Ingredients

- 1/2 cup unsweetened applesauce (low-potassium)
- 1/2 cup low-potassium yogurt
- 1/2 tsp ground cinnamon
- 1/4 tsp ground nutmeg
- 1/2 cup ice cubes

Preparation

- Combine all ingredients in a blender.
- Blend until well mixed and creamy.

Nutritional Information

- Calories: 90
- Protein: 3g
- Potassium: Approximately 80mg

Serving Size: 1 smoothie

Preparation Time: 5 minutes

4. Tropical Delight Smoothie

Ingredients

- Pineapple chunks (canned in juice, drained) of 1/2 cup.
- 1/2 cup mango chunks (frozen)
- 1/2 cup low-potassium yogurt
- 1/2 cup coconut milk (unsweetened)
- 1/2 cup ice cubes

Preparation

- Place all ingredients in a blender.
- Blend until smooth and creamy.

Nutritional Information

- Calories: 140
- Protein: 3g
- Potassium: Approximately 100mg

Serving Size: 1 smoothie

Preparation Time: 5 minutes

5. Creamy Vanilla Oatmeal Smoothie

Ingredients

- Rolled oats (cooked and cooled) of 1/4 cup
- 1/2 cup low-potassium yogurt
- 1/2 cup low-potassium milk substitute (e.g., almond milk)
- 1/4 tsp vanilla extract (low-potassium)
- 1 tsp honey (optional)
- 1/2 cup ice cubes

Preparation

- Combine all ingredients in a blender.
- It should be blended until the oats are fully incorporated and the smoothie is creamy.

Nutritional Information

- Calories: 180
- Protein: 6g
- Potassium: Approximately 100mg

Serving Size: 1 smoothie

Preparation Time: 5 minutes

6. Berry and Spinach Power Smoothie

Ingredients

- 1/2 cup fresh or frozen blueberries (low in potassium)
- 1/2 cup fresh or frozen strawberries (low in potassium)
- 1/2 cup baby spinach
- 1/2 cup low-potassium yogurt
- 1/2 cup low-potassium milk substitute
- 1 tsp flaxseed meal
- 1/2 cup ice cubes

Preparation

- Place all ingredients in a blender.
- Blend until smooth and vibrant.

Nutritional Information

- Calories: 120
- Protein: 5g
- Potassium: Approximately 120mg

Serving Size: 1 smoothie

Preparation Time: 5 minutes

7. Carrot Cake Smoothie

Ingredients

- 1/2 cup cooked and mashed carrots (low-potassium)
- 1/2 cup unsweetened applesauce (low-potassium)
- 1/2 tsp ground cinnamon
- 1/4 tsp ground nutmeg
- 1/2 cup low-potassium yogurt
- 1/2 cup low-potassium milk substitute
- 1 tsp honey (optional)
- Ice cubes (optional)

Preparation

- Combine all ingredients in a blender.
- Blend until creamy and fragrant.

Nutritional Information

- Calories: 100
- Protein: 3g
- Potassium: Approximately 120mg

Serving Size: 1 smoothie

Preparation Time: 5 minutes

8. Peanut Butter and Banana Smoothie

Ingredients

- 1/2 banana (sliced, remove potassium by soaking in water)
- 1 tbsp peanut butter (low in potassium)
- 1/2 cup low-potassium yogurt
- 1/2 cup low-potassium milk substitute
- 1 tsp honey (optional)
- Ice cubes (optional)

Preparation

- Place all ingredients in a blender.
- Blend until smooth and creamy.

Nutritional Information

- Calories: 200
- Protein: 8g
- Potassium: Approximately 160mg

Serving Size: 1 smoothie

Preparation Time: 5 minutes

9. Mocha Almond Smoothie

Ingredients

- 1/2 cup brewed coffee (cooled)
- 1/2 cup unsweetened almond milk (low-potassium)
- 1 tbsp cocoa powder (low-potassium)
- 1 tbsp almond butter (low in potassium)
- 1 tsp honey (optional)
- Ice cubes (optional)

Preparation

- Combine all ingredients in a blender.
- Blend until smooth and energizing.

Nutritional Information

- Calories: 50
- Protein: 2g
- Potassium: Approximately 50mg

Serving Size: 1 smoothie

Preparation Time: 5 minutes

10. Papaya Paradise Smoothie

Ingredients

- 1/2 cup fresh papaya (peeled, seeds removed, low-potassium)
- 1/2 cup low-potassium yogurt
- 1/2 cup low-potassium milk substitute
- 1 tsp lime juice
- 1 tsp honey (optional)
- Ice cubes (optional)

Preparation

- Place all ingredients in a blender.
- Blend until the smoothie is creamy and tropical.

Nutritional Information

- Calories: 80
- Protein: 3g
- Potassium: Approximately 120mg

Serving Size: 1 smoothie

Preparation Time: 5 minutes

CHAPTER 6

7 Days Meal Plan

Day 1

Breakfast: Spinach and Tomato with Scrambled Egg Whites

Lunch: Chicken and Vegetable Stir-Fry

Dinner: Lemon Herb Baked Chicken

Day 2

Breakfast: Oatmeal with Cinnamon and Apple

Lunch: Quinoa and Black Bean Salad

Dinner: Quinoa and Vegetable Stir-Fry

Day 3

Breakfast: Greek Yogurt Parfait

Lunch: Turkey and Vegetable Wrap

Dinner: Baked Cod with Herbed Cauliflower Rice

Day 4

Breakfast: Cottage Cheese and Pineapple Bowl

Lunch: Spinach and Mushroom Omelette

Dinner: Spinach and Mushroom Stuffed Chicken Breast

Day 5

Breakfast: Rice Cake with Almond Butter and Banana

Lunch: Tuna and White Bean Salad

Dinner: Turkey and Vegetable Stir-Fry

Day 6

Breakfast: Egg and Spinach Breakfast Wrap

Lunch: Broccoli and Rice Casserole

Dinner: Lentil and Vegetable Soup

Day 7

Breakfast: Quinoa Breakfast Bowl

Lunch: Grilled Chicken Salad with Lemon Dressing

Dinner: Salmon and Asparagus Foil Packets

CHAPTER 7

Conclusion

I found myself at the center of a journey—a voyage into the intricate world of low-potassium diets and their tremendous impact on the lives of seniors dealing with the challenges of chronic kidney disease (CKD). It's been a journey that has taught me not only about potassium levels, but also about the power of choice, resilience, and the unyielding spirit of people who have chosen this path to greater health.

As we consider the recipes, meal plans, and vital ideas presented within these pages, I am reminded that health is more than just the absence of disease; it is also the embrace of life's full potential. Each recipe is a tantalizing promise of sustenance, energy, and vigor for those who have chosen to begin on this changing path.

Throughout this book, we've learned the critical relevance of a low-potassium diet for seniors, particularly those suffering from CKD and other illnesses. We've learned about the importance of potassium, its role in the body, and the delicate balance that must be maintained to ensure our health. We've investigated a wide range of foods that provide nutrition while adhering to potassium limitations.

We've looked into the human spirit's resiliency. The experiences of seniors who have negotiated the maze of CKD with grace and tenacity are a monument to the fortitude that each of us possesses. They motivate us to be health advocates, to seek knowledge, and to make educated decisions that improve the quality of our lives.

This book is more than just a recipe collection; it is a celebration of life, a tribute to the wisdom that comes with age, and a compass pointing us in the direction of maximum health. It serves as a reminder that, no matter what obstacles we face, we have the ability to take charge of our well-being and enjoy the tastes of life.

Remember that you are not alone as you finish this book and begin your own adventure. You carry the knowledge, recipes, and inspiration to confidently and joyfully adopt a low-potassium diet. May your route be filled with tasty discoveries, better health, and the completion of your own unique, changing journey.

Made in the USA
Coppell, TX
07 October 2024